Six Steps To A Healthy Lifestyle

A Practical Approach to Improve Your Health

Michael P. O'Donnell, MBA, MPH, PhD

CONTENTS

Improve Your Odds of Success
1. Think about what is really important to you
2. Figure out how to make it less difficult?

Chapter 4: Build Skills

Evidence-based approaches triple success rates

Make a plan

Get help

Figure out your favorite learning style

Refine your goal and write down your plan to achieve it
1. Be specific
2. Be measurable
3. Be challenging but achievable

Make a commitment to a friend or family member

Build a social support network

Create a supportive physical environment

Feedback: Track your progress and make adjustments

Celebrations

Figure out what you value most

Choose celebrations that support your wellness goal and are healthy for you in general

Group competitions

Chapter 5: Form Habits

Chapter 6: Help Others

Conclusion

Author's Note

Changing your health habits is kind of a big deal. It takes time and focus. It can also produce benefits that can change your life. If you have a good plan, you can be more efficient and you can increase your likelihood of success. This book provides a framework for that plan and has six steps:

1. Get Ready
2. Measure Your Health
3. Set Goals
4. Build Skills
5. Form Habits
6. Help Others

1. Get Ready

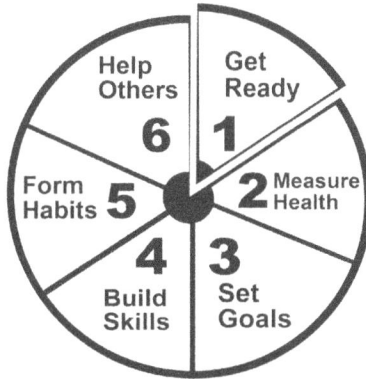

Getting ready is about reflection upon what, how much and how you want to change. It's about thinking how serious you are about changing. It is about reflecting on what is at stake and what could be. Maybe you want to overhaul your life. Maybe you want to make some minor adjustments here and there. Maybe you don't really want to change. Maybe you are not sure what you want to do. It's OK. Whatever you want to do or change is OK. It's your life. You should focus on what's important to you.

In sorting this out, think about what is at stake. Are you happy? Are you fulfilled? Do you have good relationships with family and friends? Are you productive and fulfilled in your work? Do you have a clear sense of purpose in life? Do you have a positive outlook on life? Are you able to handle daily and chronic stresses without driving yourself and others crazy? What is important to you? How important is good health to you? If you improve your health, how will that improve the things that are important to you? Are you focusing your attention on the things that are most important to you in life?

If you are overweight, what will losing 10, 20, 30, 40 or 50 or more pounds do for you? Will it make you feel better about yourself, make your clothes fit better, give you more energy in the day, stop those muscle aches and pains, or improve your appearance?

If you have a sore back all the time, or you don't have enough energy to work a full day and have fun with family or friends after work, or you can't pick up and hug your kids or grandkids because you are out of shape - what will getting in shape do for you?

If you smoke, and it makes you start each day with five minutes of hacking in the sink, or breathless when you walk up the stairs, or desperate to put a cigarette in your mouth whenever you feel stressed, see certain people or find yourself in certain places, or anxious when you haven't had your hourly jolt of nicotine, or broke because you spend $2000 a year for your pack-a-day habit, or irritated that you have to go outside to smoke when you are at work, in a restaurant, or visiting friends, or tired of hearing people tell you that your clothes, furniture and breath stink - what will quitting do for you?

How important is it to you to be around for your friends, children, parents and other family members? How important is it to see them through the milestones of life, to set a good example for them, to be strong and healthy so you can help them when they are old or sick?

These are not trick questions. The health benefits of controlling weight, quitting smoking, getting fit, managing your stress and eating nutritious foods are clear. Smoking, being sedentary or being very overweight will kill most people about 10 years early. Lack of physical activity is tied to at least a dozen serious chronic diseases. Smoking damages almost every organ in your body. Poor nutrition almost doubles your chance of dying each year. But how important are all of these things to you?

How will improving your health improve what is important to you? This question is important because making changes in your life takes time, commitment, patience, and persistence. If improving your health is not very important to you, if it will not improve your life, then you may not want to proceed any further. If it is important, you should have a sense of the next steps you need to take.

Research shows us that the *Get Ready* stage is important in making successful behavior changes. Dr. Fishbein and Aizen's *Theory of Reasoned Action* has shown us that people's intention to change is a very good predictor of whether or not they actually change. Dr. Prochaska's work on the *Stages of Change* portion of the *Transtheoretical Model* shows us that people often pass through several stages of readiness to change. These stages include *Precontemplation*, in which they are not planning to change in the next year, *Contemplation* in which they are open to change in the next 6 month, *Preparation* in which they are planning to change in the next month, *Action* in which they are in the process of changing, and *Maintenance* in which they have made the change and are actively working to maintain the new behavior. One of the keys to success in the *Get Ready* stage is to open your mind and heart to the possibility of change…change that will help you achieve what you decide you want to achieve.

2. Measure Your Health

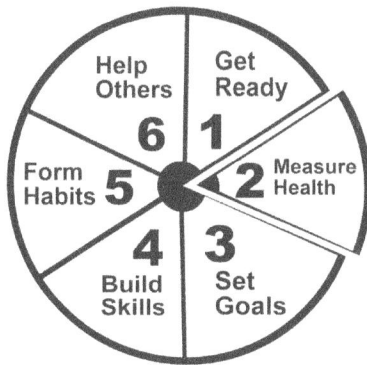

A n important next step is getting an objective measurement of your health and learning more about the link between your own lifestyle and your health.

LIFESTYLE QUESTIONNAIRE

A great way to get started is to fill out a lifestyle questionnaire. These questionnaires are sometimes called health risk assessments, or health risk appraisals, and are sometimes abbreviated as "HRAs." Lots of employers offer HRAs for free as part of a wellness program, as do some insurance companies. Check with them first because the HRA they offer may be tied into a comprehensive wellness program that can support all of your ongoing change efforts.

If you can't find a HRA at work or through your health insurance company, you should try one of the free online programs. One of the best free wellness websites is RealAge: http://www.realage.com/. In addition to providing a free lifestyle questionnaire, it includes lots of other wellness tools. Online wellness is a fast growing field, so there will be many more great sites emerging in the coming years.

Five Dimensions of Optimal Health

Many people and a growing number of scientists think of health as something much broader than just physical health. *The American Journal of Health Promotion*, one of the leading research journals in the field, defines optimal health as "a dynamic balance of physical, emotional, social, spiritual, and intellectual health." These dimensions and the types of programs that can be used to improve them are described below.

Physical Health is the condition of your body. Programs to address physical health usually focus on fitness, nutrition, weight control, quitting smoking, alcohol and drug abuse prevention, and medical self-care.

Emotional Health is the ability to cope with or avoid stress and other emotional challenges. Programs to address emotional health include employee assistance programs (EAP), stress management, and programs to enhance happiness.

Social Health is the ability to form and maintain nurturing and productive relationships with family, friends, co-workers, neighbors, and others. Programs to address social health can include training in parenting, conflict resolution, assertiveness, and other skill building areas, as well as opportunities for employees to get to know each other in fun social activities and to serve others through volunteer projects.

Intellectual Health encompasses achievements in academics, career, hobbies and cultural pursuits. Programs to address intellectual health can include job-focused mentoring and skill enhancement programs, as well as more broadly focused tuition reimbursement policies, book clubs, and cultural outings.

Spiritual Health is having a sense of purpose, love, hope, peace and charity. For some people, this is drawn from being part of an organized religious group; for others, it is having a sense of values inspired by other influences. Programs to address spiritual health can include workshops to help people clarify life priorities and set goals as well as allowing people to embrace their religious beliefs.

EMOTIONAL, SOCIAL AND SPIRITUAL HEALTH

The RealAge questionnaire focuses primarily on the physical health dimension, with some attention to the social and emotional dimensions. It does not measure spiritual or intellectual health. The connection between spirituality and health has been explored for centuries, but measurement of spirituality and health is relatively new. I am not aware of one questionnaire that measures all the aspects of this relationship, but the Authentic Happiness website offers free online questionnaires on core strengths, emotions, engagement, meaning, life satisfaction and other topics. Their website is: http://www.authentichappiness.sas. upenn.edu/

ESTIMATING BALANCE IN THE FIVE DIMENSIONS OF OPTIMAL HEALTH

One of the core messages of this book is the importance of striving for balance in the five dimensions of optimal health. To estimate balance in your life, I do not recommend a complex battery of tests. Instead, I recommend reflecting on the simple question: How balanced am I on the five dimensions of optimal health – that is, physical, social, spiritual, intellectual, and emotional health?

EXERCISE SAFETY QUESTIONNAIRE, THE PAR-Q

Exercise really IS the best medicine, but even the best medicine is sometimes dangerous for some people. For those who need to be more physically active, it is important to acknowledge that there is a very small, but real risk of heart attack and even death from strenuous exercise, especially for those with genetic conditions and those who are very out of shape.

The Physical Activity Readiness Questionnaire (PAR-Q) in the Appendix was developed by The Expert Advisory Committee of the Canadian Society for Exercise Physiology, in conjunction with the British Columbia Ministry of Health. I encourage you to complete this form to help you decide if you need to see your doctor before you start to exercise.

The benefits of exercise far outweigh the risks, and this caution is not intended to keep anyone from being more physically active. For those who are out of shape, continuing to be sedentary is far more dangerous than being active. Unless you have a medical condition that prevents it, or specific advice from your doctor to not be active, adding a little more walking around your house or at work is good for everyone.

HEALTH SCREENING

Health screenings come in all shapes, sizes, and prices. Some are free through health fairs, employer or health insurance company programs, and others can cost thousands of dollars in the form of executive physicals. For the purposes of setting wellness goals, I recommend the tests below, preceded by a 12 hour water-only fast. In addition to giving you a good sense of your health needs, getting baseline measures in these areas can help you see the progress you make as you improve your health habits. You can see dramatic improvements in all these areas (except height of course) if you quit smoking, eat more nutritious foods, and exercise more regularly.

Blood pressure and resting heart rate
Glucose
Triglycerides
Cholesterol (Total, HDL, LDL & Ratio)
Height, weight
Waist and hip measurements

Collectively, these tests measure metabolic syndrome. Metabolic syndrome is the likelihood you will contract diabetes, have a stroke, or develop heart disease sometime in the future. If you have abnormal values in three of the five areas, you have metabolic syndrome. The specific tests change slightly from time to time. For example, we used to think it was sufficient to measure height, weight, and waist circumference to get a crude sense of obesity. Now we realize we should determine the ratio of the waist to the hips. Also, for those with high glucose levels, additional tests might be required to detect diabetes or the likelihood of getting diabetes. These tests are simple and inexpensive to perform.

If you are going to get a more complete exam, make sure two things are true:

1. Your exam should include tests that are most important for your age, gender and health condition. Three of the best sites for information on these tests and other preventive services are below.

- Canadian Task Force on Preventive Health Care: http://canadiantaskforce.ca
- US Preventive Services Task Force: http://www.ahrq.gov/clinic/uspstfix.htm
- American Academy of Family Physicians: http://www.aafp.org/

These web sites are a bit complicated and their content may be difficult for the average person to understand. The simplest strategy is to ask your doctor which tests you need before the exam.

2. Make sure you have a clear understanding of how you will use the results of your exam to make changes in your life. Some executive physical programs focus far too much on extensive and expensive lab tests and too little on how to interpret and act on the results.

TALK TO YOUR DOCTOR

If you have any serious medical conditions or answered yes to any of the Questions in the PAR-Q, you really should talk to your doctor about your plans to improve your health. You may find that he or she can be a great partner in helping you to get data, set goals, build skills, and monitor your progress. Do your homework before you go. Complete the lifestyle questionnaire before you see your doctor and give some thought to the goals you want to set.

Once you have the information you need on the link between lifestyle and health, you are ready to move to the next stage: setting goals to improve health.

3. Set Goals

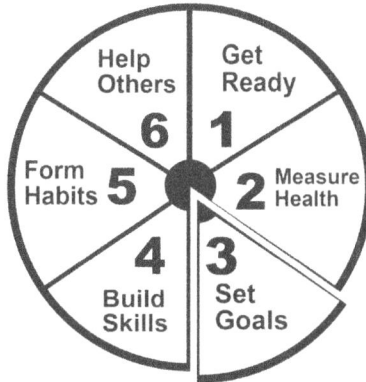

Setting goals is important to success in any area of life. If you don't know what you want, how do you know the first step to take to get there? How do you know if you are making good progress? Setting goals is also one of the most important things you can do to improve your health. In fact, two of my colleagues, Dr. Ron Goetzel and Dr. Cathy Heaney, discovered this when they reviewed all the research that had been published on comprehensive workplace wellness programs. They discovered that success rates were double in programs that included personal goal setting.

Goal setting is part science and part art. Science tells us a few things:

1. Set challenging goals, but make sure that you are committed to the goal and that the changes you need to make are under your control. Research tells us that setting challenging goals increases performance 52%-82%.

2. Set specific goals. General goals like "I will do my best to improve my health" are not likely to have much impact. Setting specific goals increases performance 42%-80%. A specific goal states what, when and how much you will do - for example, "I will walk 30 minutes a day at least four days a week."

3. You can improve your level of commitment by reinforcing the importance of the goal in your mind, making a public commitment, finding leaders who inspire and actively support you, and being actively involved in setting your own goals. Enhancing your sense of self-efficacy can increase your commitment as well. (See discussion on enhancing self-efficacy later in the book.)

4. Get feedback on your goals on a regular basis. When people realize they are falling short of their goals, they increase their effort.

5. Set short- and long-term goals. Short-term goals allow you to measure progress on a regular basis. This allows you to celebrate successes and reinforce your efforts or make adjustments in your approach or your goals before you get off track. Long-term goals provide inspiration.

6. Setting goals helps us in several ways. Goals help us focus our attention on the behaviors that are most likely to make a difference, increase the amount of effort we are willing to exert, and help us be persistent when we are fatigued.

To succeed in setting a wellness goal you can achieve, you need to focus on three basic questions: What, Why and How?

WHAT TO FOCUS ON FIRST?

Most people have a long way to go to improving their health. In fact a national study by Quanhe Yang published in the March 28, 2012 issue of the *Journal of the American Medical*

Association found that only 1% of Americans had all seven of the seven health metrics important for avoiding heart disease. These include not smoking, being physically active, not being over weight, eating a nutritious diet and having normal blood pressure, cholesterol and glucose.

What changes should you think about and which ones should you change first? Should you try to change a lot of things at once or focus on changes one step at a time? If you have a major crisis in your life, like a life-threatening injury, AND you can devote a big chunk of your time to making changes, some experts have found that changing everything at once can be successful. This strategy often requires lots of support from experts, family and friends and ALWAYS requires lots of motivation. Immersing yourself in a residential treatment program or spa where you can focus 100% of your time and have easy access to experts, might be the best way to achieve a whole life change. However, long-term success in a major or minor change always requires learning skills and forming habits in your normal surroundings, so you can stay on track month after month, year after year.

Making small changes, one at a time, is a more successful strategy for most people. The key is to match your goals with your effort. If you want to lose 100 pounds through lifestyle change, it is certainly possible, but it will probably require adding an hour of physical activity to almost every day of your life for three years, learning how to cook in a whole different way, and replacing the junk food in your life with fruits, vegetables, whole grains and beans. Are you willing to make that level of change? If not, its certainly OK, but you are not likely to lose the 100 pounds, and you should focus on goals you can achieve by making the changes you are willing to make.

A good place to start is to list all the health changes you think would improve your health based on what you learn in the "Measure Your Health" step….then focus on Why.

WHY DO YOU WANT TO CHANGE?

It's your life. It's a free country. You shouldn't do anything you don't want to do, and you should do as much of what you want to do as much as possible. Of course we all have to be realistic. Most of us have to work to pay the bills, and hurting other people puts us in jail or worse. Short of those limits, you SHOULD focus on what you want, and you should align your efforts with what you want.

So, what is important to you? What is going to make you the most happy and fulfilled?

Is health important to you? It is important to me. I want to be healthy because I want to be healthy. I know: this is irrational circular logic. I think about health every day. Some people might say I am obsessed about it, although I do my best to appear laid back about it. I don't think I fool too many people. Over the last 40 years I have learned that I am a little weird. I admit it; I confess in public to the world. I am a health nut. I used to be focused primarily on my physical health. I worked out at least three hours every day for almost 10 years of my life. When I was in graduate school at University of California, Berkeley, most students were obsessed with learning, getting A's, and getting great jobs. I was the weird one who scheduled my academic classes around classes in gymnastics, weight lifting and tennis. On top of that, I usually ran seven miles a day, played intramural water polo, and at the end of the day rode my bike two miles up a steep hill to get home. I was also a vegan, and I did not eat any refined sugar or other junk food for four years. It worked. My body fat was less than 5%. My total cholesterol was 81, my resting heart rate 55, and I had more energy than anyone I knew. But I was a little weird, and I gave up a lot by focusing so much on fitness. I could have spent more time learning in school. I could have spent more time with friends. I could have spent more time helping others. I don't regret my focus on fitness. I loved every minute of it, and I am still passionate about health, but I have broadened my focus. I strive for balance in the five dimensions of optimal health: physical, social, emotional, spiritual, and intellectual. Before college, I was focused on the spiritual dimension. When I was newly married and had young kids, I was pretty focused on the social dimension. For the past 15 years, I have focused a bit too much on the intellectual dimension, and am trying to focus more on the social dimension. My point is not to talk about me; it is to acknowledge that physical health is not the number one priority for everyone all of the time.

Sure, other people focus on their health and they value good health, but for most people, health is a means to an end, not the end in itself. They focus on their health so they can feel good every single day, so they have enough energy to pursue a demanding career, so they have enough energy to work all day and not feel exhausted in the evening when they are with friends and family, so they can be a good role model for their kids, so they can play with their grandkids or be alive to see their kids and grandkids grow, so they can feel like they are a responsible person, so they can honor their God, so they can look good, so they can go skiing, play golf, climb mountains, explore the world...so they can do the things that are important to them.

Health is kind of like money. Some people focus on making a lot of money because they value money itself. They want to amass lots of money. They like to count it. They focus their time and energy on amassing as much money as possible. Now let's be honest, most people do like money, and most people wouldn't mind having more than they have right now, and most people will put in time to make money. But most people want money to allow them to do the things they want. They certainly want money to be able to buy the basics...food and shelter. They may want money to be able to go on vacation, buy toys, give gifts, put their kids through school, and save for retirement. Some people want money to impress other people, or to feel good about themselves, or to be able to do good in the world by giving lots away. For others, money is just a by-product of working hard and doing well in a career.

Most people have a general sense of their priorities in life, or at least know what makes them feel good. However, it is very easy to get caught up in raising a family, pursuing a career, and just surviving in the rat race....and lose track of our priorities. Several times in this book I have encouraged you to take a step back, think about what is most important to you in life, write down your priorities, and reflect on how well your daily activities get you closer to what is most important to your in life. The next step, from a health enhancement perspective, is to figure out how to tie your priorities with things that are good for your health. If you do that, health will take care of itself.

CONNECTING WHAT AND WHY WITH HOW TO CHANGE

Different people approach goal setting in different ways. Analytical, engineering types (OK, I admit it, I fit in that category) like to spell everything out in great detail. If you can tolerate this approach, it is probably going to be the most effective. Unfortunately, most people can't put up with all the detail and prefer a less structured approach. The less structured approach is the focus of the remainder of this book.

The first step is to answer three questions.
1.   What are your priorities in life?
2.   What are your health needs?
3.   In what ways can changes in your health habits help you achieve your priorities in life?

1. What are your priorities in life?

I have asked this question hundreds of times to thousands of people on six continents over the past two decades. The responses are remarkably consistent. Family, health, and work are usually the top three, usually in that order. Faith and peace are the next most common responses. For simplicity, I lump family and friends into the same category. I also lump work, earning a living and learning into the same category. So what are your priorities in life?

2. What are your health needs?

The self-reflection you did in the *Measure Your Health* stage gave you a good sense of the changes you need to make to improve your health. The study by Quanhe Yang showed us that 99 out of 100 of us need to exercise more, eat better, lose weight, quit smoking or lower our blood pressure, cholesterol or glucose. Do you need to change one of these? Maybe you need to drink less alcohol, or floss your teeth, or stop using dangerous drugs, or better manage your stress, or get more regular medical check ups. Make a list of the health habits or conditions you need to change.

3. In what ways can changes in your health habits help you achieve your priorities in life?

This one is the key. If you can figure out how changes in your health habits will help you achieve what is important to you in life, you will be forever motivated to change these health habits.

I have explored this connection with hundreds of people. A young engineer in Detroit told me that his top priorities were to be a great engineer, fall in love, and get married. His typical routine was to work until 8:00 pm, go to a downtown bar to eat dinner, and try to meet women. He ended up eating greasy hamburgers and chips, drinking lots of beer, spending lots of time in smoke filled rooms (this was before the era of smoke free bars), and staying up so late that he was tired at work most days. He found himself starting to smoke on and off, gaining 20 pounds, and getting involved with women who did not share his ambitions. Eventually, the quality of his work started to slip and he received his first negative job rating. After some reflection, coaching, and experimentation, he discovered that he could fulfill his desire to meet women by joining a co-ed running club and taking cooking lessons held in the early evening near his home. This forced him to leave work at a reasonable time and allowed him to get to bed early, wake up naturally in the morning, and be more alert at work.

A prominent doctor at the Cleveland Clinic told me that he came to the Clinic because he wanted to work with and be among the best clinicians in the world. His priorities in life were the health of his patients and clinical breakthroughs. He derived great pleasure and satisfaction from his work and did not want to work less. However, he was starting to feel run down and was less productive at work...which is why he wanted to talk to me. He was willing to start lifting weights and add 40 minutes of brisk walking to his daily routine only because he discovered that it reduced his back pain and gave him more energy so he could work longer.

A nurse at the Cleveland Clinic told me that she was devoted to caring for her patients. She was loved by her patients and admired by her co-workers because she extended her heart to each of her patients every day. Unfortunately, this drained her emotionally and physically. She found herself scarfing down junk food during short breaks all day because she did not have time to eat a good lunch. She was exhausted at the end of the day and found herself being impatient with her kids and husband. She stopped having friends over because she did not have time to clean her house and she was embarrassed that it was a mess. That was the final straw. She signed up for a ballroom dance class with her husband so they would have dedicated exercise-focused time together two days a week. She also started a routine of active playing or walking with her kids every day after work. Her favorite change was a new family tradition of engaging the whole family in household chores every weekend.

START WITH SUCCESS

The next step in the How process is to figure out what to change first. My overall advice is to choose a goal you are likely to achieve. If you are successful in achieving this first goal, it will help give you the confidence you need to take on the next goal.

Ask the questions below about all the possible health changes you might make.

1. How important is it to YOU?
2. Are you ready to make this change NOW?
3. Have you done this BEFORE?
4. How DIFFICULT will this change be?

1. How important is it to YOU?

Why do you want to make this change? Is it important to you, or are you doing it for someone else? There is nothing wrong with starting to think about making a change because someone else brought it up. People who quit drinking often do it because their family and friends confront them and tell them it is necessary, but the ultimate motivation has to come from within.

Robin, one of my friends from Texas, found herself in this situation. Her mother, a co-worker, two sisters, and a best friend confronted Robin on her drinking. Her mother told her she would always love her but could no longer see her when she was drunk. Her co-worker told her she admired the creativity Robin brought to the firm they ran together but could no longer put up with the missed deadlines and embarrassment caused by Robin's drinking, and she would sever their partnership if she did not stop drinking. Robin's sisters told her they were concerned about the environment in which Robin was raising her young daughter and told her she might lose custody to her divorced husband. Robin did go into treatment and has been sober for 15 years. Her family and friends pushed her into this decision, but she did not quit drinking for them. She quit because she wanted to raise her daughter in her own home, continue her successful business partnership, and maintain loving relationships with her family.

John, one of my co-workers, quit smoking because it upset his son. Every morning, John would start the day hacking in the sink to spit up the phlegm that had accumulated in his lungs over the night. As John lit up a cigarette, his son came into the bathroom crying that he was scared that John would get more and more sick and die. This shocked John into seeing what could happen to him if he kept smoking. He quit not because his son begged him to, but because he wanted to be a good role model to his son, and he wanted to be alive to see his son grow.

It is probably easier to illustrate this point by sharing some failures. Sally decided to lose weight to make her boyfriend think she was more attractive. She switched to a vegetarian diet, joined a health club and lost 30 pounds in just three months. It was a lot of work but she felt more attractive than she had ever felt. Two weeks later, her boyfriend broke up with her to be with someone else. She was so depressed that she stopped working out and started eating junk food. She gained 40 pounds.

Laura decided NOT to work out because her husband put so much emphasis on being fit. She did not want to have a cute fit body because she wanted her husband to love her for who she was, not what she looked like.

The point is, you are more likely to be successful in making and sustaining a change if the change is important to you and if it is going to enhance parts of your life that are important to you.

2. Are you ready to make this change NOW?

Earlier, I talked about the concept of stages of readiness to change developed by James Prochaska. Think about each of the changes you are considering. Choose the changes you are ready to make now. Come back to the others when you are ready.

3. Have you done this BEFORE?

One of the best predictors of success in the future is success in the past. If you used to run on a regular basis a few years ago, you can probably start running now without a lot of difficulty. You may not be as fast as you used to be, and it may take months to get past the painful stage, but you know what to do and how to do it, so it will be relatively easy. You also know how good it feels once you get in shape, so you know what to look forward to. If you never ran before, if you were never athletic in high school or college, it will be a lot more difficult to start now. The great news is that you have the chance to feel better than you have ever felt before. You have heard people talk about it…the runner's high, the endorphins. You can have this for the first time in your life, but to get there, you will probably need more help.

4. How difficult will it be to make this change?

If you exercise on a regular basis and you are trying to add a stretching routine to your workout two days a week, that's pretty easy and you can probably succeed. You need to learn how to do the stretches by reading up or working with an instructor. You need to figure out where it will fit in your routine, if you will add more time to your workout, or if this change will require you to drop another exercise. You also need to practice it enough times so that it becomes a habit. You need to think through these steps and focus your attention on this small change, but it should be very achievable.

On the other hand, if you have been overweight most of your life and you figure out you need to lose 100 pounds as fast as possible, you have a lot of work to do. You should definitely take the PAR-Q in the Appendix. You will probably need to see a doctor to determine if you have diabetes, high blood pressure, or any other health problems that could be aggravated by being more active, or if you have other heath problems that may be causing your weight gain. You will need to figure out a way to add an hour of physical activity to your life every single day. This activity could be 20 minutes of walking before work, two sets of 10 minutes of walking during work, and 20 minutes of active chores at home in the evening. You can also increase your physical acitivity in a more organized way; for example, you could join a health club, take aerobics classes, or get a personal trainer. As long as it adds up to an hour a day of activity, it does not matter very much *how* you become more active. You also need to change the way you eat forever. Diets don't work. Actually, they usually work in reverse. You do lose weight at first, but your body gets used to living on fewer calories, so when your diet is over and you go back to your original eating habits, you gain the weight back. Many people gain more weight than they lost, and more of it is fat than before. If you have been overweight all your life and you want to lose 100 pounds, you also have to learn how to eat in a whole new way. You need to learn what foods to eat, where to buy them, how to cook them, how to handle family and friends, and how to deal with going out to eat. You also need to learn about controlling your portion sizes, not sometimes, but every time you eat. If you stick with these changes, you will lose the 100 pounds, but it might take three years. And you will have to maintain this lifestyle the rest of your life to keep the weight off. Are you prepared to do that? If yes, go for it. If no, set a less ambitious goal that you can achieve. Taking 3 years to lose 100 pounds probably seems like a long time, especially if you make drastic changes in your exercise and eating habits. From another perspective, 3 years is actually very fast when you realize that it probably took 20 or 30 years to gain this weight. It may be more realistic to set a goal of losing 50 pounds in 3 years, then set a new goal of losing 50 more pounds in the next three years.

With long time frames of several years, it is important to set short term goals and celebrate them as they are reached. The great news about weight loss is that every pound you lose improves your health. For example, losing 7% of your body weight can reduce your blood pressure and reduce the chances you will get diabetes. For a 200 pound person, this means losing only 14 pounds. See Chapter 4: Build Skills for more details on setting short term goals and celebrating milestones.

If you find that you are having trouble falling asleep at night because of work, you might find yourself in one of two situations. You might have a great work situation, but you have the habit of rehashing problems that happened at work that day. You might be able to break this cycle by finishing your work day with a five minute review of what went well and not well during the day, writing short notes about what you will do the next day to address the problems....and leaving it on your desk at work, so your can address it the next day when you return to work. This brings temporary closure to the problems. The next step might be to start a ritual that ends your work day and starts your private evening. It might be doing some sort of physical exercise. It also might be playing with kids, seeing friends you enjoy, doing public service, or reading a good book. The point is to fill your evening with something positive and different from work. Before you go to bed, you might think about two or three things that went well during the day and think about why they went well. This exercise has two benefits. First, it makes you feel good about your day, and it helps you relax so you can fall asleep. Researchers in the field of positive psychology have also found that this exercise improves your sense of happiness for an extended period of time. If you find yourself thinking about work in bed, shift your focus to thinking about your family or an upcoming event you are excited about. Building these new routines into your life may take several months. Making these sorts of changes requires discipline, but it is not overwhelming because you have all the factors under your control.

On the other hand, you might find yourself in a very stressful job situation. You might have a job you are really not qualified to do well, or you may be asked to do things you feel are unethical. You might have a boss who makes unreasonable demands or treats you with disrespect. Your organization might be going through layoffs or unnerving restructuring. Handling these situations will take much more work. Is your strategy going to be to learn how to cope with this difficult situation, help the organization change, or leave your job? Helping the organization change may take years, and it may never change. You may need to go back to school to get more education. You may need to apply for a new job. You may need to go through a period of unemployment. Are you ready and able to make that level of change?

In thinking through the level of difficulty, think about three factors:

1. How much of the solution to the problem is under your **control**? Are you in a position to make all the necessary changes to correct the problem?
2. Do you have the **support** you need to make the necessary changes? Are your family, friends, co-workers, supervisors, and others ready to provide the help and resources you need to make the change?
3. Do you have the **skills** you need to make the changes you want to make? If not, do you know where you can find books, websites, coaches or other experts who can help you gain the skills you need to make the changes you want to make?
4. Does your level of **commitment** match the level of effort necessary to make the change?

IMPROVE YOUR ODDS OF SUCCESS

After you think through all of these issues, you may find yourself conflicted. You may decide that you are likely to be successful flossing your teeth on a regular basis but you really, really should quit smoking even though it will be more difficult to succeed. You have two choices: start with the goal you are more likely to achieve (flossing your teeth on a regular basis) or improve your odds of being successful in quitting smoking.

You may also discover that you are not likely to be successful in changing ANY of the things you are thinking about changing, but you really think you should make an effort. You have two choices in this case also: you can give up and do nothing; or you can improve your odds of being successful.

If you want to improve your odds of success, you can do two things:

1.   Think about what is really important to you.
2.   Figure out how to overcome obstacles.

1. Think about what is really important to you

Sometimes people convince themselves that some goal (eg. getting a certain job, meeting a certain person, quitting smoking, losing weight, etc.) is not important to them because they think it is unachievable. To see if this is true for you, think about each of your possible health goals (eating nutritious foods, exercising regularly, quitting smoking, losing weight, better managing stress, etc.) and then think about what your life would be like if you achieved that goal.

If it is quitting smoking, think about taking a deep breath of fresh air without coughing. Think about walking up three flights of stairs without wheezing. Think about not having to wonder when you are going to have a heart attack or get throat, mouth or lung cancer. Think about not having to worry if your breath smells bad when you talk to people. Think about not having to clean your furniture, car and clothes to get out that smoke smell. Think about having an extra $2000-$4,000 to spend on clothes, vacations, or your family every single year. If you are a man, think about not having to worry about erectile dysfunction. Think about not having to stand outside in the rain or cold to satisfy your addiction. Think about not being seen as a bad influence on kids.

If it is losing weight, think about how you will feel about yourself when you look in the mirror. Think about fitting into those clothes you haven't worn in years and being able to find clothes that fit and look great in all the stores.

Think about not having to worry that people don't like you because of the way you look. Think about being able to be on your feet all day without getting exhausted. Think about not being obsessed with food. Think about not worrying you will get diabetes, or heart disease, gall stones, or knee and ankle problems.

If it is getting fit, think about having enough energy to work all day and play in the evenings. Think about not having aches and pains in your knees and back. Think about actually being able to FEEL a sense of wellbeing throughout your body. Think about being able to eat more of the things you like to eat without gaining weight. Think about being productive the entire day.

If you can visualize yourself having achieved your goal, if you can assume for the moment that you will be successful in achieving that goal, and if you like how that feels, then you can get a more accurate sense of how important that goal is to you. Using this strategy will help you figure out which goal is most important to you without being confused by your fear of failure in achieving that goal.

2. Figure out how to make it less difficult

Sometimes people are reluctant to attempt a change because they think they will fail. In some cases, they have a realistic sense of the difficulty. See Chapter 4: Build Skills for specific strategies to make change less difficult. In other cases, they are just talking themselves into failure. The good news is that you can talk yourself out of failure. Scientists call this enhancing self-efficacy. Self-efficacy is the belief that you can perform a specific behavior. The behavior can be giving a speech, writing a report, building a house, exercising every day, not smoking, etc. People with high self-efficacy are more likely to attempt adopting a new behavior, more likely to follow through with all the steps necessary to be successful, and less likely to relapse to the old behavior. The opposite is true for people with low self-efficacy. There are four dependable ways to enhance self efficacy: 1) practicing, 2) watching others, 3) coaching, and 4) understanding your body. Each of these strategies is discussed in the box on page 26.

More details on setting goals are in Chapter 4.

Enhancing Self-Efficacy

Practice (Mastery). The most powerful way to enhance self-efficacy is perform the new behavior successfully. Breaking the new behavior into small steps can makes it easier to be successful on each step, and success on the first step will make you more confident that you can achieve the next step. Your confidence will be even greater if you are persistent in overcoming challenging obstacles. People who recognize the important role they play in their progress have an even greater sense of self-efficacy. The opposite is also true; if you fail repeatedly, you get discouraged and lose your confidence.

Watching others (Vicarious learning). If you see other people being successful in performing the new behavior you want to perform, especially people who are similar to you, it increases your confidence that you can perform the behavior as well. Your confidence increases more when you see others encounter and overcome challenging circumstances.

Coaching (Verbal persuasion). Your confidence also increases when people encourage you in your efforts, especially when they express their confidence that you can succeed in achieving realistic goals. People you respect, including coaches or teachers, can be very influential in this way.

Understanding your body (Physiological feedback). When you understand the physiological reactions of your efforts to change, they are less threatening to you and less likely to discourage you. For example, if you know in advance that feeling a physical craving for cigarettes is a very normal part of the quit process (and can even be seen as a first step in the process), you are more likely to remain committed to quitting. Similarly, if you know in advance that feeling out of breath or sore is very normal for people who start to exercise that have been sedentary, you will be less likely to quit.

All of this thinking can be a bit cumbersome, but it is very important to your ultimate success because it forces you to focus on what is most important to you. Once you decide what you are going to focus on first, you are ready to build new skills. The first part of building those skills is to set specific goals.

Take A Health Break

Is this getting a little overwhelming? Are you tired of THINKING about getting healthy, and want to get started ACTING healthy RIGHT NOW? Good. Put down this book and go do it right now. If your goal is to get fit, go take a 20 minute walk. If your goal is to improve your eating, go eat a fresh piece of fruit or a raw vegetable. If your goal is to manage your stress, close your eyes, take deep breaths for 5 minutes, and think about someone you love. If your goal is to lose weight, make a promise to yourself right now that you will not eat any junk food the rest of the day and take a 20 minute walk to reinforce that promise. If your goal is to quit smoking, promise to not have another cigarette today. Any time you are tempted to have a cigarette, do one of the healthy habits above: take a walk, take deep breaths, or eat a piece of fresh fruit.

From now on, any time you want to stop thinking and start doing, put down this book, choose any of these health breaks, and DO IT.

4. Build Skills

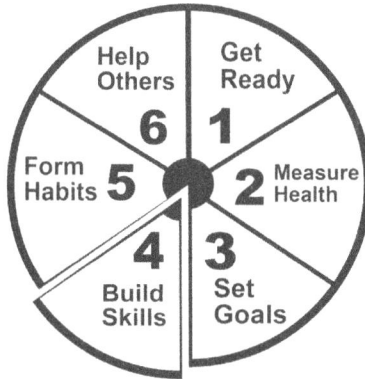

If you were going to learn a new language, what would you do? The best strategy would be to immerse yourself in a culture that speaks that language, so you could hear people speak, watch how their lips and face move as they express each of the words and phrases, and learn about their customs so you could better understand the underlying meaning of phrases. You would also need to learn grammar rules and vocabulary, using books, tapes, or a language coach to help you. Most importantly, you would need to practice, practice, practice.

If you were going to learn how to play soccer, you could start by watching others play. You would need to learn the rules by reading manuals and talking to people. At some point you need to meet people who play soccer so you can play with them. To get good, you need to learn the individual moves, how to dribble with your feet, how to trap (or catch) a ball with your feet or any other part of your body (except your hands), how to pass or take a shot on goal. If you want to get really good, you need to learn how to dribble past a defender with speed or finesse, how to kick a ball that is six feet off the ground by doing a modified back flip, or put spin on the ball when you kick it, so it changes direction in mid air to go over or around a defender. Having the right books, a coach, and patient teammates really helps during this process. Eventually, you need to internalize the rules and know them without thinking, so you don't go off-sides, commit a foul, or get yourself thrown out of the game. To play at the highest level, you need to master the individual moves so you perform them instinctually when an opportunity presents itself. You also need to learn mental toughness so you can keep playing at full speed when you are exhausted, hurt, or way behind.

Changing a health behavior is a lot like learning a new language or playing a new sport, except it is usually a lot harder, because you need to break habits you have formed over decades of time. If you could immerse yourself in a culture that supports your new lifestyle, it would be a lot easier, but that is not an option for most people. So you have to find or build subcultures that can support you and teach you how to resist the influences of the cultures that have supported the unhealthy habits you have learned and practiced for decades. Think about it: you have indeed honed these habits through decades of practice, practice, practice. They are part of you. You perform them without thinking. They are comfortable. They are part of your identity. You need to learn new habits, and learning new habits usually takes months and sometimes takes years. In the case of quitting smoking or chewing tobacco, you also have to overcome a chemical addition to nicotine. Weight loss is more complicated because you cannot just quit eating - you need to learn how to eat differently.

If you are going to be successful in changing your health habits, you need to build new skills.

EVIDENCE-BASED APPROACHES TRIPLE SUCCESS RATES

Eighty percent of smokers say they want to quit, and 40% try to quit every year. Most of them try to quit "cold turkey." They do it on their own without any guidance. They often shun assistance. As my neighbor used to say, "I don't need any help. I have quit smoking lots of times." Of course he was never able to stick with it. In fact, only 5% of people who quit on their own are successful in quitting. Smokers who use scientific methods to quit are three times more successful than those who do not; in other words, 15% are able to quit if they have help in doing so. Using several approaches at once is also a good idea; for example, smokers who combine behavior strategies (self study books, web programs or telephone, face to face counseling) with drugs (nicotine replacement therapy, Wellbutron, or Chantix) are five or six times more successful, and 25%-30% are able to quit smoking.

Admittedly, a 25% success rate means a 75% failure rate. People fail because it is very hard to quit smoking. For most people, quitting smoking means changing a habit they have practiced for decades. Any habit you practice year after year is hard to change. On top of that, smokers build their daily routines and social lives around smoking. They have a cigarette to help them wake up. They have a cigarette with their cup of coffee. They have a cigarette when they are feeling anxious, or to celebrate the end of the day, or when they get in their car. They have a cigarette when they see certain friends. The typical smoker has 10 or 15 routines or friends that trigger them to smoke.

On top of that, cigarettes are manufactured to cause people to become physically addicted to nicotine. Smokers are physically hooked, just like a heroin addict. Considering all of these factors, it is not surprising that 95% of people

Grampa and his Pipe

My grampa Pat loved his pipe. At the end of each day, he would sit down in his recliner chair, dip into the can of tobacco he stored within reach, pack his pipe, light a match, draw in a long breath to ignite the tobacco, then let out a long breath. He let go of all his cares with that breath. It was the end of his workday, and the beginning of his evening. He was proud of his pipes and he wanted to share that tradition with his grandson. He taught me how to clean out the pipe bowls and shaft with a pipe cleaner, how to pack the tobacco so it would not burn too fast or too slow. We had rituals built around his pipe smoking. He taught me how to go to the drug store and ask "Do you have Sir Walter Raleigh in a can?" When the clerk said "Yes", I would say 'Better let him out!" then run down the aisle giggling hysterically while my Grampa looked at me with pride. For nearly five years, every Christmas and birthday present for Grampa was related to his pipes... pipe ashtrays, ties, tie clips, pipe cleaners, tobacco travel pouches, cans of tobacco. One of his favorite gifts, something he kept his entire life, was a Christmas card I made out of a piece of cloth and framed. I embroidered his favorite things on the cloth...a train car, a dump truck and a pipe. How could Grampa ever quite smoking his pipe? It would be turning away from an important ritual he shared with his grandson.

who try to quit on their own fail. The good news is that people who use the best scientific methods are 5 to 6 times more successful.

MAKE A PLAN

What is your plan for success? How are you going to learn the rules of your new game? How are you going to learn the moves? Who are you going to practice with? Who is going to coach you? How are you going to immerse yourself in a culture that models the behaviors you want to adopt and nurtures you through the process?

GET HELP

Most of us need help when we make a big change in our lives. You may be different, but probably not. This book helps you understand the cognitive process of change and the kind of structures you need to be successful, but it does not tell you the clinical details and specific techniques on how to exercise, how to prepare food, how to manage stress, how to quit smoking, etc. You probably need help on those details. The key is to match the complexity of the change you want to make with the amount and form of help you draw upon. If you want to change something simple, like starting to floss your teeth every night, you can probably get a brochure from your dentist or simple instructions on the web. If you want to lose 100 pounds, you need more help.

FIGURE OUT YOUR FAVORITE LEARNING STYLE

What is your favorite way to learn? Do you like to read books, surf the web, talk on the phone, take a class, meet with a personal coach? Figure out how you learn best, and use that approach to gather all the detailed information you need.

The next step is to set a specific goal, but you really need to educate yourself before you can set an informed goal.

REFINE YOUR GOAL AND WRITE DOWN YOUR PLAN TO ACHIEVE IT

Once you have a clear sense of what you need to do, write it down in the form of a goal. Your goal should be specific, challenging but achievable, under your control, and measurable. You should write it down and share it with a friend.

Be specific

- If you want to quit smoking, set a quit date within the next month.
- If you want to get fit, what kinds of physical activity are you going to do? What type of activity

can you add to your daily life? What type of formal exercise program will you start? When and where will you do it? Who will you do it with? How will you learn the best exercise for you? Will you improve your flexibility, your muscle strength, your endurance, or all three?

- If you want to improve your nutrition, how will you learn the best foods to eat? Where will you buy your food? How will you prepare it? What will you do when you travel, eat as a guest in someone else's home, or go out to dinner?
- If you want to lose weight, state a specific goal weight, with a weekly weight loss goal of 1 to 2 pounds. Specify what you are going to DO to achieve that goal. How much physical activity are you going to add to each day? What foods are you going to eat to reduce your calorie intake?
- If you want to better manage your stress, how will you figure out what is causing stress in your life and how will you learn how to eliminate or cope with those stressors? What techniques will you practice and when will you practice them?

Be measurable

State your goals in a way that allows you to measure progress. Include health outcome goals like pounds and inches lost, fitness levels achieved, and so on. Also include behavioral goals like the amount of time you spend exercising and the foods you eat.

Be challenging but achievable

If you set an unreasonably difficult goal, you are likely to fail. Conversely, if you set a goal that is too easy, you won't be challenged to put forth the effort, you wouldn't see the impact, and you are also likely to fail. When I was in graduate school, I had a girlfriend who was smart, beautiful and basically wonderful in every way you could imagine. She was not very athletic, and she thought this was a threat to our relationship. Remember, I was the obsessed fitness nut with 5% body fat, and this was my definition of health.

She knew how much I valued fitness and she also saw how much pleasure it brought me. She decided she was going to show me she knew....without telling me. With virtually no background in running, and no coach, she decided she would run the San Francisco Marathon, which was just 4 months away. Within a month, she had reached 10 miles on her longest runs...double what she had ever run in her life before that month. That's when she revealed her plan to me with pride. I was impressed with what she had accomplished, and in awe of her goal, partly because I had never run a marathon myself. Unfortunately, she quit the next week because she was exhausted every day and her legs hurt all the time. If she had set her sights on a 10K race, she would have achieved her goal of running the first race of her life, and may have eventually worked up to a marathon.

You can also err on the side of setting a goal that is too easy. My high school buddy decided he wanted to lose weight, but he heard that moderation was the best approach. Gary was 38 years old and had gone from 170 pounds to 220 in the 20 years since he graduated from high school. He decided to lose the 50 pounds at twice the rate he gained it...5 pounds a year. He figured out that a teaspoon of sugar was worth 15 calories and walking slowly for 5 minutes was worth 45 calories. He knew he had to build something into his life that would become part of his routine. He realized he had two consistent habits that were not likely to change: one was drinking a cup a coffee with two teaspoons of sugar every morning as soon as he woke up, and the other was watching the evening news after work. He figured out that coffee with two teaspoons of sugar was 36 calories. He decided to drop from two teaspoons of sugar to one, for a savings of 15 calories a day; over 10 years, this was worth 54,750 calories or 15.64 pounds. He also decided to pace in front of the television for the first five minutes of the evening news; this was worth 164,250 calories or 46.93 pounds, for a total of 62.57 pounds in 10 years...12 pounds to spare. From one perspective, this was great thinking, because it showed how very small changes can make a big difference over time, and it helped him understand how he gained 50 pounds in 20 years. He did great at first. In the first month, he used one teaspoon of sugar in his coffee every single day.

He also paced for the first five minutes of the evening news every single day. At the end of month, he stepped on the scale, and as expected, saw no difference. Theoretically, he lost half a pound but the scale was not precise enough to show the weight loss. He decided to get a digital scale and start the next month. One day, his wife's boss dropped by after work. Six o'clock rolled around. Gary reached for the clicker to turn on the news and started to stand up. His wife glared at him, horrified that her boss would see her neurotic husband pacing in front of the TV set. Gary put down the clicker and eased back into his chair. A few days later Gary was traveling to Seattle on business and strolled into a new coffee shop. He ordered something called Frappuccino, Mocha, Whipped & Tall. The rest is history. He now weighs 230 pounds.

MAKE A COMMITMENT TO A FRIEND OR FAMILY MEMBER

Dr. Steve Nissan is a prominent cardiologist from the Cleveland Clinic. When he was 12, he asked his dad (also a doctor) how he could smoke cigarettes despite overwhelming evidence that it was deadly. His father made a commitment to his son to quit on the spot and never smoked again. When you make a promise to your child, most people will do everything they can to fulfill it, even if it means great personal sacrifice. You can build on this principle by making a sincere commitment to your child, your spouse, another family member, or a friend to stick with your behavior change goal. If you are not willing to make this type of commitment, maybe you are not serious about making this change and you should rethink it. If you are ready to make this commitment, it will increase your resolve to be successful.

BUILD A SOCIAL SUPPORT NETWORK

Ross, Karen, Pat, Ian, Dennis, and Russ. I got up at 5:00 am to swim 3 miles, 4 days a week for 8 years with these knuckleheads. We lifted weights the other days. Most days, it was hard to get out of bed. Most days, the water was cold when we jumped in. Everyday, we pushed each other so hard we were out of breath most of the workout. There was not much time to talk. We swam interval workouts, which meant we usually had 3 to 20 seconds between reps, and one or two minutes between sets, but over the years, the seconds and minutes added up and we got to know each other pretty well. I was so tired after most workouts I usually had to take a nap later in the morning. We nursed each other through injuries. We helped each other train for races. We all had demanding jobs. We all traveled a lot. But we all went to the pool when we were in town because we did not want to let each other down. I can remember many days when I wanted to just roll over and go to sleep, or get an early start on my work, but I went to the pool because I did not want to be the one who made someone else swim alone because I did not show up.

My dad was an alcoholic but he was not a drunk most of his life. In fact, he did not have a drink in the last 45 years of his life. He decided alcohol was ruining his life, and he quit. Many people try to quit and fail. If you could ask him why he was successful, he would tell you one key reason is the commitment he made to a group of people he saw every Wednesday night. He and my mother went to this group almost every week for 45 years...more than 2000 times. When they lived overseas for four years, they found a new group. When he traveled, he would find a local group. Over time, his primary group become much more than a support group to help him stay sober; its members have became some of his closest friends in the world.

Dean Ornish, MD, cardiologist and best-selling author, created a comprehensive lifestyle change program that has been successful in reversing heart disease, something traditional medical practice has never achieved. PET scans of his patients have documented regression of myocardial perfusion abnormalities and coronary artery stenosis... which means that heart problems reversed themselves and arteries that were clogged became unclogged. His program includes exercise, nutrition, stress management, weight control, and tobacco treatment. It consists of weekly meetings for five years. It is a scientifically sound program led by a very talented staff, but if you ask Dr. Ornish why it works, he will tell you it is the social dimension created by this group of people who see each other every week for years and become a community.

I came to the same conclusion after interviewing members of this community. One of the men I spoke to was a prominent San Francisco attorney named John who had a heart attack several years before I met him. He was overweight, inactive, smoked cigarettes, and ate a horrible diet whenever he was out of the house. His wife was fed up. She loved him, but she didn't want to see him die. She told him she would divorce him if he did not join Dr. Ornish's program. He thought the program was bunk, but he adored his wife and went with her every week. He did a great job of changing his diet, quitting smoking, and exercising on a regular basis, but he was still a hard driving type A, and hated sitting in a circle with the group to discuss stress and other lifestyle issues. During the group discussions, he usually sat with his arms folded tight, resenting the time wasted by the group and silently ridiculing other group members who were talking about the changes they were making in their lives. Two years after he joined the program, he was listening to a new member talk about how hard it was to not get mad every time his boss asked him to go on a business trip. As a boss who often told his employees to travel, John could identify with this, so he uncrossed his arms and leaned forward to give this young man some great tips on how to handle his boss. When he finished talking, no one spoke. Everyone in the group was looking at John in disbelief because this was the first time he had said anything of substance in two years...after nearly 100 meetings. John told me his eyes welled up, and tears rolled down his checks. He realized it took him two years, but he was finally ready to embrace the valuable messages embodied by this program. He was finally willing to accept the members of this group as his friends. After that night he was one of the most engaged members in the group. If he had not been part of the group for several years, he would have never let down his barriers to let the message sink in, and he would still be a hard driving SOB (his words).

Goal setting is probably the most important factor in the beginning of a successful lifestyle change effort, but social support is probably the most important factor in sustaining lifestyle change.

CREATE A SUPPORTIVE PHYSICAL ENVIRONMENT

What parts of your environment support your goals and what parts detract from them?

Chris was a close friend who went to graduate school with me at the University of California, Berkeley. When he started graduate school, he moved from San Francisco across the Bay to Berkeley. By the end of the first year, Chris had gained 10 pounds. We couldn't figure out why. He ate the same food and kept up the same exercise routine. We realized the difference was the hills of San Francisco. Lack of parking and steep hills make driving difficult in San Francisco, so Chris walked every place he went. Chris's apartment in San Francisco was on a long steep hill. To get any place, he had to walk up that hill. He walked up the hill to work every day. On weekends, he walked up the hill to go to a ball game, to go to the park, to go grocery shopping, to visit friends. Driving was easy in Berkeley, so he drove a lot more often.

I lived in Seoul, South Korea for a year as a visiting professor. I was not able to find a swim team to work out with, but I found a great replacement...hiking. Seoul is a great place to hike because there are dozens of big hills and small mountains, within the city limits. I lived on one of the big hills. My wife and I hiked up 1000 feet to the top almost every day. This took about 20 minutes up and less down and was always a pleasure. The small mountains around Seoul had a vertical climb of about 4,000 feet in addition to several miles of approach. A hike to the top and back typically took 5 to 6 hours of pretty hard work, and was one of the most exhilarating things I have ever done. I hiked these mountains with two buddies who run marathons on a regular basis, Bill Whitmer and Judd Allen, and both agreed it was a very challenging workout. The biggest payoff, however, was the reward at the top of the mountain. First, you saw the panoramic view of the city, then you reached a centuries old wall built to defend the city from foreign invaders.

Finally, you were offered a cup of tea and an invitation to rest at an ornate Buddhist temple. By the time I left Korea, I felt that hiking had become my number one sport and looked forward to hiking in the United States. I moved back to Michigan, which has no mountains and few big hills. I have not taken a hike in Michigan in the 16 years since I left Korea because my physical environment does not support it.

Reid Ewing, a professor at the National Center for Smart Growth at the University of Maryland, examined the relationship between "connectivity", which is the opposite of sprawl, and body weight, in a study that involved 425,000 people in all the counties of the United States. Manhattan is the most "connected" county in the US because of the dense population, cross streets and alleys that provide direct access to lots of great places, easy access to public transportation, side walks, and close proximity of places to live, work and play. It is very easy to live and work in Manhattan without a car. In contrast, Geauga County, outside of Cleveland, Ohio, is impossible to get around without a car because of its rolling hills, spacious estates, and its long, winding country roads with few sidewalks, bicycle right-of-ways or places to walk on foot. In fact, Geauga County is tied for last place in the nation in connectivity. Reid discovered that the weight of the people living in an area was predicted in part by "connectively." For example, the people of Geauga County weighed an average of 6.3 pounds more than the people of Manhattan, and were 29% more likely to have high blood pressure. He found that people who lived in the 25 least "connected" counties walked an average of 191 minutes per month compared to 254 minutes for those in the most connected communities.

If you live in a place that gives you easy access to places to be physically active, especially places that are fun and alluring, you are far more likely to be physically active.

Similarly, if you have access to nutritious food, you are more likely to eat nutritious food. I was a volunteer at the Berkeley Free Clinic while I was going to graduate school in public health. My job was to talk to people who came in for help. One day, a young African-American woman came for help. She was concerned that her kids were eating too much junk food. I felt like I could help this woman. I had studied nutrition informally for more than four years before I decided to become a vegan. I told her about all the fruits, vegetables, grains, legumes, and nuts I ate, where I bought them and how I prepared them. She was very patient with me, and congratulated me on my nutritious diet. Then she told me they did not sell fresh produce in the liquor store. I said "Huh?" She told me the liquor store was the only place in her neighborhood that sold food, and, all they sold on most days was canned spaghetti and potato chips. She acknowledged that she could take the bus 45 minutes each way to shop where I shopped, but what would she do with her 3 kids? She couldn't leave them at home alone. Needless to say, I learned more that day from her than she learned from me. This woman was motivated to feed her children nutritious food, but she did not have easy access to it. Many, if not most, inner city neighborhoods have the same problem.

Your environment does indeed shape your behavior. When it pushes you in a positive direction, take advantage of it. When it pushes you in a negative direction, be aware of this and avoid it. If you are organized and determined, you can shape your environment to support your health goals.

Although I am no longer a vegan, I am still a vegetarian and I have a ridiculously healthy diet. That does not mean I am never tempted. If there is no junk food around me, I don't miss it, and I don't buy it at the store. However, I also have little discipline at the point of consumption. Every once in a while, especially when I am watching TV, I have a craving for junk food. I scrounge through all the cupboards looking for a hidden stash of sweets. If my wife has done a good job of hiding them and I don't find them, I am pleased to have a banana. If not, I am liable to gobble up a hand full of sweets. Knowing this, I alter my environment to eliminate the junk food. I also avoid making the purchase of junk food when I am at the store in a rational mindset.

FEEDBACK: TRACK YOUR PROGRESS AND MAKE ADJUSTMENTS

Regular reflection on your progress can help you stay on track and give you the chance to make adjustments when you get off track. It also gives you a great opportunity to celebrate your successes.

A good way to track your progress is to break your long term goal into shorter term goals or milestones. I suggest you think in terms of five milestones

Milestone 1:   Make a commitment to change.
Milestone 2:   Develop a change plan.
Milestone 3:   Learn the skills you need to change. This might include learning how to perform specific cardiovascular exercises, how to plan and prepare nutritious foods, how to react to stressful situations differently, how to wean yourself from tobacco, and so on.
Milestone 4:   Try out each new skill for the first time.
Milestone 5:   Practice each of your new skills on a regular basis.

If you are NOT successful in reaching each of these milestones, pause and reflect on the possible reasons why you are having trouble. Of course, your ultimate goal is losing weight, improving your fitness, quitting smoking, etc. It helps to break those goals into milestones as well. If you are trying to lose 50 pounds, you might break this goal into 5-pound loss increments spread over two years. If you are trying to quit smoking, you might think in terms of the individual days you are smoke free, then whole weeks, and whole months, and eventually years. If you are trying to improve your fitness, you can think in terms of being able to walk, run or swim a certain distance (or at a certain speed) or being able to lift a certain weight.

CELEBRATIONS

Reaching each of these milestones is cause for celebration. Celebrating progress helps most people recommit to their goal. Frequent celebrations are fine. You do not need to wait until you have achieved your ultimate goal. Celebrate after each PART of the 5 milestones. Celebrate after EACH of the skills you learn, EACH time you try to practice a new skill for the first time, EACH time you are successful at making the skill a habit. Celebrations also do not need to be elaborate. In some cases, leaning back, taking a deep breath, and acknowledging your progress to yourself is enough. Reflecting on your progress several times that day or mentioning it to a good friend can be satisfying, but you should also think of some more elaborate celebrations. I encourage you to consider the relative impact of extrinsic vs. intrinsic incentives in the sidebar in planning your celebrations.

Extrinsic versus intrinsic rewards

Extrinsic rewards come from external sources. Money is a common extrinsic reward. Intrinsic rewards come from within. Having a sense of satisfaction, feeling fit, and having renewed energy are common intrinsic rewards that come from improved health. There is some risk in focusing too much on extrinsic rewards because it distracts people from the numerous intrinsic rewards that come naturally from improving health.

Whenever possible, I like to draw on intrinsic rewards. Intrinsic rewards have two main advantages: First, they are readily abundant to us if we know how to tap into them, and second, they usually work better.

It is becoming more common for employers to charge lower health plan premiums for employees who practice healthy lifestyles or meet certain health goals. We have discovered that financial incentives are very effective in motivating employees to participate in programs. They motivate employees to be involved in health screenings, to participate in health education or skill-building programs, or to engage in just about any activity. Unfortunately, there is very little evidence that financial incentives change health behavior. We suspect this will be true for most extrinsic rewards, unless they are very large. Another problem with extrinsic rewards is that people sometimes start to think that receiving the extrinsic reward is their ultimate goal, and they lose sight of the intrinsic reward of improved health. When they stop receiving the extrinsic reward, they might be tempted to stop practicing the new, healthier behavior. This is an important issue when organizations are trying to motivate individuals to achieve certain outcomes, but it is probably less important when people are planning their rewards and celebrations for themselves.

If an employer's goal is to attract and retain the healthiest employees, it probably makes sense to offer incentives or other discounts for healthy behaviors, because healthy employees will feel rewarded and be likely to join and stay. However, unhealthy employees will be likely to feel punished and be more likely to leave. If the employer's goal is to stimulate employees to improve their health, it makes more sense to reward them for things that are completely under their control, like participating in programs.

FIGURE OUT WHAT YOU VALUE MOST

Different people like different types of rewards. Some people love public recognition, others are embarrassed by it. Some people feel honored to be congratulated by a high level boss or celebrity, others feel it is not genuine because those people have no connection to the achievement. Maybe you like to treat yourself to a movie. Spending time with a good friend or carving out time to read a good book might be a great reward. One of my special pleasures is to take a long hot bath. Choose rewards that are valuable to you.

CHOOSE CELEBRATIONS THAT SUPPORT YOUR WELLNESS GOAL AND ARE HEALTHY FOR YOU IN GENERAL

Many cultures around the world equate celebration with splurging on food…usually high fat, sugary food…or by drinking lots of alcohol. Why not? It's fun and it feels great… at first. It also leads to all the health problems we have been discussing. Splurging on food might not be a great way to celebrate your wellness milestones, especially if you are trying to lose weight.

GROUP COMPETITIONS

Group competitions are very popular, for understandable reasons. They are a great way to make health goals visible. They are also a great way to build social support around health goals. Competitions around losing the most weight or running or walking the furthest distance are very common. They often involve everyone contributing a small amount of money and the highest achiever winning the jackpot. These competitions have two problems. First, when the jackpot is large, they sometimes cause people to go to extremes that can be dangerous. For example, people might be motivated to lose weight by eating virtually no food, drinking no water, or by vomiting up food. Losing too much weight too fast is dangerous in the short term and often results in weight gain in the long term. This risk can be minimized by forming teams who collectively compete for the prize and measuring weight loss for the whole group and not counting weight loss above a certain amount, maybe 2 pounds per week. This approach increases the number of winners and also decreases the amount of the jackpot received by one person. Another problem with competitions is that winners feel good, and losers feel bad. Winners attribute their success to their efforts, but losers often attribute their failure to their inability to make an effort. This can reduce their self-efficacy and discourage them from trying to lose weight in the future. The damage can be minimized by rewarding all participants in some way and by helping everyone understand that they are making progress if they are working to change their health habits and they can be successful if they follow a plan like the six step process in this book.

5. Form Habits

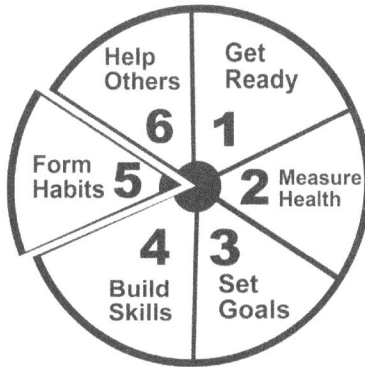

Dieting doesn't work. Virtually everyone who goes on a diet to lose weight, fails. They fail not because they don't lose weight. In fact, most well-conceived diets do produce weight loss...for a few weeks or months. Diets usually fail because most people revert to their old eating habits when they reach their weight goal...and they regain their weight. People succeed in losing weight and keeping it off when they change how they eat...forever. The same is true for getting fit. Working out for a month or a year gets you in shape for that month or year, but when you stop exercising, you eventually get out of shape. The key to successful long term health behavior change is to build your newly formed health skills into habits you practice every single week, and in most cases, every single day.

Peter, one of my former work colleagues, decided to get in shape shortly after we started working together. He started by walking...first 10 minutes a day, then 20, then 30, and eventually 60 minutes a day. He then added a two hour walk on the weekends. The weight started peeling off quickly. Peter was a big man, about 6'2" and 240 pounds. Over a period of 6 months, he lost 25 pounds and reached 215 pounds. Next, he worked on his diet, adding lots of fruits and vegetables, getting rid of most of the meat and sweets, and the pounds continued to drop. He lost 10 more pounds, reaching 205. He became an excellent cook, and really enjoyed serving healthy food to his family, but hit a plateau by the end of the year. Despite this great progress, Peter was a little discouraged. He wanted to reach his college weight of 190. I asked him to describe his workout plan and his eating habits. He was keeping up the heavy workout schedule and said he ate his very healthy diet almost every day. I asked him what he meant by "almost." He said he liked to indulge in a big dinner and lots of dessert on special occasions, like his birthday. I said that was a little self-defeating, but was probably OK if he did it just on his birthday. Then he said it was not just on HIS birthday, it was also on his kids birthdays and his wife's. It was also at weddings, and other parties. He also acknowledged it was hard to refuse extra servings when he went out to a friend's house for dinner...and it was hard to find nutritious food in most restaurants...plus the portions were big. His work forced him to travel at least six times a year. It was pretty easy to figure out the problem. We added up all the "special occasions" and they totaled nearly 60 days a year - or one out of every six days. We also estimated that Peter ate more than double his normal calories on those days. We stopped working together at that point, so I don't know if he ever made any further progress.

When you add a new positive behavior to your life, it often takes months of diligent discipline to keep practicing the new behavior. An addictive behavior, like smoking cigarettes, can take as much as five years of diligent discipline. Most of the time you feel the immediate rewards of your new behavior, and that keeps you going, but remaining disciplined is draining work for most people. If you can build the new behavior into your routine, you take away the need to discipline yourself.

Your routines change over the span of a lifetime, and you need to adapt with these changes in routines to form new habits around exercise. In high school, I exercised in varsity sports practices. Sports practice was always after school. In college, I exercised whenever my various gym classes were held. The changing schedule of classes did not matter because my habit was that I always took gym classes. When I graduated, I joined a swim team that worked out in the morning before work, usually at 5:30 am. Learning to get up at 5:00 am was tough. It took me months of pain to make that adjustment, but after a few years the habits were ingrained: 30 years later, I still wake up at 5:00 am without an alarm and I need my morning fix of exercise or the day just does not feel right.

When I was 31 and working as a health promotion director in a community hospital, our finance director told me walking was the best exercise. He was middle-aged, probably 58. I remember being polite to him but not taking him very seriously. Walking was for old people and was probably not enough, even for them. I was in peak shape at the time. I was buff and had little interest in walking. Boy, was I wrong - walking IS great exercise, for just about everyone. True, if you want to get buff, you need to walk a lot and you need to complement it with mid-body and upper body strength exercises as well as flexibility exercises, but walking is so powerful because our bodies are built for walking. Some people are able to run marathons all their lives, but after a while, running wears down the knees and ankles of most people. Our bodies are built to walk and most people can do it all their lives. It works for people of all fitness levels. Coach potatoes and people who are completely sedentary can stand up and take a five minute walk…today. People who already exercise but want to lose a few more pounds can add walking to their daily routine to shed those pounds. A 140 pound person who walks an additional mile a day, five days a week can lose or avoid gaining 6 or 7 pounds in just one year. The other beauty of walking is that you can do it any place. You can walk in your neighborhood and chat with your friends. You can stroll through a mall and window shop. You can cut your grass. You can play in the yard with your kids. You can go for a hike in the park. You can walk while you meet with colleagues at work. You can walk up the stairs instead of taking the elevator. You can also break it into short bouts of 10, 5 or even a few minutes each. If you decide to take the elevator instead of the stairs, you can pace until the elevator arrives...although some people may think you are a little weird.

One of the main reasons we have an obesity epidemic in the United States is that we have engineered activity out of our lives. When I was a child, I walked to school every day. My children took the bus or were driven. People used to live in complete neighborhoods that allowed them to walk to the store, to a movie or restaurant and sometimes to work. Most communities are so spread out that a car is necessary to go most places. Most communities are built for cars. Rather than walk to the corner for the bus or subway, we back out of garages, drive to work and often park in the basement of the buildings we work in. We use remote clickers to turn on the TV, send emails at work rather than walking down the hall, and surf the net to do research rather than brose through the library. These advances have significantly improved our productivity, but they have also made us sedentary.

When I started working in a new job at the Cleveland Clinic, I was a bit overwhelmed by the huge campus of our main hospital, which spans 21 blocks by 3 blocks in the middle of Cleveland, Ohio. I also saw a great opportunity to build lots of walking into my work day by scheduling meetings all over campus. This gave me the opportunity to learn our campus and meet the many people I would be working with. I found myself spending up to 40 minutes a day scrambling from one meeting to another. I added a little game to this scrambling. My days were packed, so I usually had to walk as fast as possible to avoid being late for a meeting. This was often a challenge because the halls were usually packed. We had 16,000 employees and 20,000 visitors on the campus in a typical day. I started imagining I was a football running back, looking for holes to run down the field. As I approached a crowded section of a hallway, I would look at the flow of people walking to discover which path would get me through the fastest. When I saw a "hole", I would accelerate through it. Of course I had to maintain the appearance that I was a professional and be careful to never brush by someone, especially a frail patient. This became a pastime I would look forward to.

My secretary told me she felt sorry for me as I was always in a rush. Little did she know that I was dashing out to play imaginary football.

When I decided to become a vegetarian in college, I really had to make only one small change. I had to sign up for the vegetarian food cafeteria at Oberlin College. It was a little awkward getting to know new people to eat with, but it was not hard to stick with eating vegetarian food, because that's all that was served. When I graduated from college and started cooking for myself, I had no trouble sticking with my vegetarian diet because it was a core ethical value for me. However, it was a big adjustment learning to shop and cook. I had spent my high school years in Korea in the late 1960's, which was a developing nation at the time. Food was sold at an open farmer's market, with many small venders for each type of food spread over blocks and blocks. The shopping process took several hours. On top of that, the market was far from home and we did not have a car available for shopping trips. Of course, there were no packaged foods, and each piece of food had to be scrubbed with boiling water. The gas stove did not always work and it exploded more than once. We had eight kids. Food preparation was literally a full time job and we had a cook who was responsible for this work. The bottom line is that shopping in a grocery store and preparing food was a completely new experience for me. I started out eating at friends' houses, and I quickly learned that I was not very good at disciplining myself at the point of consumption. If you hold a brownie under my nose, I am likely to bite your fingers off as I inhale it in one bite. Actually, maybe I am exaggerating; that sounds more like my dog. I quickly learned that the best way to have nutritious food in my house was to purchase only nutritious food at the grocery store. That way there was never junk food around when I craved it. What a luxury to discover that I was able to go to a grocery store that sold all the food I could possibly want. I found a great store that sold nutritious food, was staffed by really nice people, and attracted really nice customers. My new fun habit was to go see these really nice people while I shopped every Saturday morning. When I got married, everything kind of fell apart. I offered to continue to cook, but my wife really did not like the incredibly nutritious but even more boring meals I prepared. To me, food was fuel. To her, food was pleasure. She took over shopping and cooking. She has a bit more discipline about inhaling junk food than I do, and she wants this stuff around the house, so she buys it when she shops. Thirty years later, we still have not figured this one out completely. She still buys the junk food, but she hides it. When I have a craving, I know it is someplace in the house, so I rummage through every cupboard, closet, drawer and alcove until I find it. Over the years I have mellowed a bit. I have learned how to resist my cravings most of the time, and have recognized that the time I have to spend to find the hidden treasure is not worth it...but it has taken more than 20 years to make this shift. For me, changing and managing my environment to exclude the junk food is a more efficient solution to eating nutritious foods.

I had the same experience with flossing my teeth. I liked the idea of flossing because it was a good way to clean out small bits of food. I usually flossed when I had food stuck between my teeth and two other times a year: the day before each of my twice annual dental checkups. My dental hygienist explained that flossing was indeed good for clearing out foods toothbrushes could not reach, but the more important function was to remove the plaque collecting between the teeth. Of course plaque leads to cavities. She predicted I would lose at least half my teeth by the time I was 60 unless I started to floss every day. I struggled to discipline myself to floss every night before bed and failed, until I moved the floss from my bathroom drawer to the edge of the sink. Seeing it on the edge of the sink reminded me to floss when I brushed my teeth before bed and it became a habit. Now, when I don't floss my teeth before bed, my mouth feels yucky and does not quite feel right until I floss it.

When I try to form a new habit, I try to look for opportunities to practice it in my daily routine. If I am trying to learn a new word, I look for chances to use in conversation. When I am trying to add a new stretch to my routine, I do it when I am having a conversation or waiting for a meeting. I always look for opportunities to add a short walk, or just add some activity to my day. If I am in a boring meeting, I stand up and get a drink, or walk to the bathroom. When I am on a long telephone call, I put the phone on speaker and mute and walk around my office. I am now trying to add more walking meetings to each of my days. In my last job, we had buttons that say "Meeting in Progress" in bold letters. We would wear these when we wanted to have a walking meeting. The buttons make it clear we are working and not just goofing off, but more importantly, they publicized the idea that you can add physical activity to work and still be productive.

For me, an important part of spiritual health is being aware of the world, or being mindful. I can look at a rock and kick it out of my way, or I can imagine the diversity of minerals it contains, and the enormous pressure required to fuse those minerals into a composite and the centuries of water, wind and tumbling required to smooth its surface.

When I walk by a building, I can turn my head and forget it, or I can imagine about all the people and creative energy required to produce it…architects, designers, carpenters, masons, electricians, plumbers, furniture makers, seamstresses, on and on. I can think about each of the materials used to build it, where they came from, how they were transported, the processes used to manufacture them, the work conditions of the people who produced them. When I eat a raspberry, I can swallow it in one gulp, or I can put it in my mouth and wait several seconds before it starts to dissolve and its juices flow across my tongue. I can roll it around on my tongue and sense different tastes… sweet on the tip, tart on the edges. I can think about how it emerged from a seed in the ground and whether the seed was planted intentionally or just fell to the ground in another berry. I can think about all the different organs, chemicals, and processes my body will subject it to as it is transformed from a tasty food in my mouth, to viscous liquid in my esophagus, and an assortment of minerals, fiber, vitamins, and waste transported throughout my body.

Being mindful is about appreciating the people around me and about the many opportunities I have. To be mindful with people, all I have to do is take a minute to really listen to someone…anyone. It can be an employee. It can be a salesperson. It can be a neighbor. It can be a patient. It is not difficult to see so much good in just about anyone.

You can see how much they love their kids, or how hard they have worked to earn what they have achieved, or the creative skills they can share, or how much they help others every single day. It is not hard to see the pain they carry and the challenges they are struggling to work through. When I am mindful, it is kind of like exercise. It gives me a burst of energy that often lasts the whole day. I have so many opportunities to be mindful throughout the day.

Looking for these opportunities gives me a double bonus. First, it really does help me find ways to add new habits to my day, and I get the benefit of practicing that new behavior. Second, it shifts my focus from trying to be compliant, trying not to be "bad," to looking for ways to be successful or good. Each time I find an opportunity, I pat myself on the back, and it reinforces the new behavior.

6. Help Others

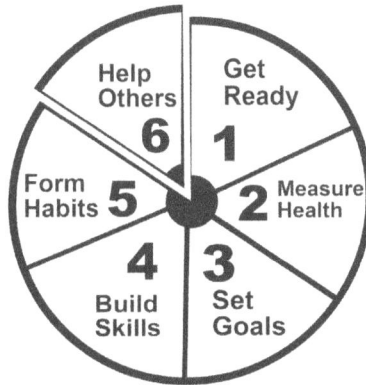

The final step in the health behavior change process is to reinforce your new health habit by helping others who are trying to form the same habit. You can serve as a mentor, organize a support group, participate in a planning committee, become an expert leader, whatever works best for you. When you help others, the immediate benefit is that it feels good. The bonus is that it also increases your commitment to your new health habit because you want to be a good role model. The double bonus is that it gives you another way to make your new habit part of your regular routine.

One of the central tenants of Alcoholics Anonymous (AA) is to help others who are trying to stay sober. This is called serving as a sponsor. The sponsor helps a new member get their bearings when they first join an AA group, and helps them through the process of staying sober. You call your sponsor when you are tempted to have a drink. The sponsor helps you understand that he or she has had the same temptations and helps you believe you can make it through this difficult period. In psychology terms, they are helping to enhance your self-efficacy by being a positive role model. I saw my father serve as sponsor to dozens of people over his lifetime. He also had a sponsor who helped him.

Valerie, one of my coworkers at the *American Journal of Health Promotion,* started taking aerobics classes to stay in shape. The regular class schedule made her work out on a regular basis and the excellent instructor helped her learn how to do the most effective exercises without getting injured. She found that she picked up the steps easily and people started asking her for help. After several months, she decided to become a certified aerobics instructor. Valerie has been teaching classes for more than a decade. Now she gets paid to do what she loves to do…teach and exercise. Aerobics has become an important part of each week of her life.

Sandy was a two-pack-a-day smoker for 20 years. She started smoking in college and had planned to quit when she graduated but discovered she was addicted and could not quit. She tried to quit five times over five years but was never successful. She decided to quit for good when she caught her 13-year-old son smoking one of her cigarettes behind the garage at her home. The next day, she called the American Cancer Society for help, and enrolled in one of their quit smoking courses a week later. Two weeks after that, she had her last cigarette. Sandy was committed to stay smoke free forever but she was tempted to smoke every single day. She joined a support group of ex-smokers and really appreciated being able to discuss these challenges with people who understood what she was feeling. Sandy helped form several new support groups and finally became a certified quit-smoking instructor. She has helped hundreds of people quit smoking. She is a great instructor because she understands what it is like to be addicted to smoking. Whenever she is tempted to start smoking now, she reminds herself that she needs to be a good role model for the smokers she is trying to help quit.

I was on the track team on and off in high school and college but had never run consistently year-round. When I moved to Berkeley California to go to graduate school, I discovered the joy of going for runs through the hills above the Berkeley campus. I used to start at the gym and run up the fire trails to the top of the hills to be greeted by a panoramic view of the San Francisco Bay. Running solo was exhilarating most of the time but very hard on long runs. During a workout at the track, I meet Marty Dicker, a graduate student in exercise physiology. We decided to start the Berkeley Runners Club and it grew to several hundred members. We organized races, matched up running partners, helped dozens of people start running and train for races, and spawned many friendships. I met dozens of friends and running buddies and they kept me running until I moved out of town.

I have listed *Helping Others* as the sixth and final step to a healthy lifestyle in this book, but there is really no final step. I like to draw the steps in a circle, because health behavior change is really an ongoing process. When you are successful in achieving one change, that is a good time to reflect on your progress, renew your commitment to the changes you have made, and get ready to tackle the next health behavior change. It is also effective to reflect on your health and start the process every year, maybe on your birthday, the anniversary of a wedding, the illness of a dear friend, or the beginning of the new year.

Conclusion

The good news is that following this six-step process and applying at least one of the strategies described within each of the steps will help you be more successful in starting and maintaining the lifestyle changes most important to you. My guess is that you will be at least twice as successful, and probably more than four times as successful...but each person is different, so it is hard to say for sure. That's the good news.

The great news is that improving your lifestyle, especially if you focus on what is most important to you, will improve the quality of your life and your personal sense of wellbeing in ways you have never imagined.

I wish you well.